Fat Losing

Book One: The Psychology of Fat Fighting

"Waste Mis-management leads to Waist Mis-management"

Gino Arcaro

Fat Losing
Book One: The Psychology of Fat Fighting

Author: Gino Arcaro
Website: www.ginoarcaro.com
email: gino@ginoarcaro.com

Jordan Publications Inc.
Canada

Editor: Matthew Dawson
Design: Shelley Palomba

Arcaro, Gino, 1957
ISBN 978-1-927851-01-2
http://www.ginoarcaro.com
Printed in Canada

Gino Arcaro's Story

I started lifting as a dysfunctional 12-year-old, trying to overcome my obesity. Lifting transformed my life physically and mentally. I have been lifting for over 43 consecutive years, 100% natural. I lift almost every day. It's part of who I am and it will always be, but it doesn't define me.

At 18, I started my policing career. A few years later, I became a SWAT team officer and then at the age of 26, a detective. At the same age, I accepted the head coach position at a high school, a decision that began a lengthy volunteer coaching career. I wrote my *SWAT No-Huddle Offense* and *Defense* manuals, (and recently published them) explaining the systems I had created and refined throughout 40 seasons of coaching football at the high school, college and semi-pro levels.

After 15 years, I left policing to teach law enforcement at the local college. During the next 20 years, I became a bestselling academic author, writing 6 law enforcement textbooks that are used in colleges throughout Ontario. Also during that time, I earned a Master degree, an undergraduate degree, and Level 3 NCCP Coaching certification. Then, in 2001, I opened a 24-hour gym called X Fitness Welland Inc. The gym continues to enjoy success in its second decade of operations. *eXplode: The X Fitness Training System* is a book I wrote that explains my workout system, based on 40+ years of lifting.

In 2010, I left teaching to make the literary transition to motivational writer. My first book, *Soul of a Lifter* was published in 2011. Since then, I've added several books. *Blunt Talk* is the name of a series I'm writing dealing with everything from fat loss to interrogation. *Soul of an Entrepreneur* is another series written to enlighten business owners – current and potential. In the series, *4th and Hell,* I tell "David vs Goliath" tales about my Canadian club football team playing in the United States. When my first granddaughter was born, I wrote, *Beauty of a*

Dream and the following year, I wrote *Mondo piu Bello* to commemorate the birth of her cousin.

I am motivated in my writing by my belief that we all have a potential soul of a lifter. We are called to lift for life. We can lift ourselves. We can lift others.

Keep lifting,

Gino Arcaro

Preface

I'm not selling a quick, overnight solution to obesity. I'm not selling a 15 or even 30-day solution. I'm not selling a diet. I'm not selling supplements. I'm selling H.E.L.L. – **H**eavy **E**xtreme **L**aborious **L**ifting – physically and mentally. I'm selling the absolute truth about losing fat. I have evidence to prove it has worked out.

However, before that, it's important for me to share with you the following before you continue:

Item 1: The title of my series is Fat *Losing*, not Fat *Loss*, because I believe that *losing* is a habit, whereas *loss* happens only once. *Loss* is temporary. *Losing* is a chosen lifestyle. *Losing* has to become habitual to win the fight. The *Losing Streak* is the top secret to staying in top shape.

Item 2: One of the worst frustrations you can experience in life is struggling with fat. Left unchecked, fat-fighting can consume you. The good news is that a good fight has a good side – it's out-of-the-ordinary, so it motivates you. The bad news is that fat-fighting can be exhausting. But you *can* win. Never let an one tell you that you can't win; especially yourself. Getting in top shape and staying there is one of life's most rewarding challenges.

Item 3: Your worst enemy isn't fat, or the struggle, or the fight, it's your mind. Your mind is the biggest obstacle keeping you from getting in the shape you want. Win the battle of your mind, and you will lose fat. That's how you keep the losing streak going for as long as you want. Keeping the losing streak alive prevents fat from making a comeback. It's all completely possible if you commit to *changing your mind.* Science has proven that the mind quits long before the body does.[1] By nature, the

---

1   University of Zurich (2011, December 5). How muscle fatigue originates in the head. ScienceDaily. Retrieved February 11, 2012, from http://www.sciencedaily.com / releases/2011/12/111205081643.htm

mind is not a hard worker, unless trying to convince the body *not* to work. The psychology of fat-losing is the single-most important element of fat-fighting. Losing the battle of the mind is the main reason why people quit working out, why people quit eating right, and why people quit fighting fat.

Item 4: I am a natural fat-fighting expert. I have 55 years of hardcore fat-fighting experience. I know exactly what it's like to *be* obese, and what it's like to *not be* obese. I know the feeling of being in the very *worst* shape, and the feeling of being in the very *best* shape. I was an obese, dysfunctional 12 year old during an ancient time, long before working-out, personal trainers, strength coaches, and supplements became fashionable. Now, I fight fat every day of my life. If I don't, I will become obese again. I'm on a 43-year fat-losing streak. I have never become obese again since I developed the proper mindset, but I *have* fallen behind on the scoreboard. Fat has made several comebacks that I challenged with a strong proactive offensive and defensive plan; a game plan that never failed to work out when I put my *mind* to it. I changed my obesity by a conscious decision to change my life radically. I started working out when I was 12, and I have never stopped. I changed my entire nutrition lifestyle, and I have never reverted back. I coached myself. I still coach myself. It's an endless workout-in-progress, but it's all worked out because I put my *mind* to it.

Item 5: The hardest concept I've ever had to teach and coach is how to get out-of-shape student-athletes into ordinary good shape, and then into the extraordinary shape needed for high risk anything. I have coached thousands of athletes; both women and men. The majority were male student athletes trying to play the highest-of-risks sport – football. Many more were female and male college law-enforcement students who wanted to work in one of the highest-of risks profession – policing.

The biggest challenge I've had is convincing them to change their *mind* about fitness. None of my students started as elite athletes or professionals. They developed through intense, consistent exercise – an amount of work that had to be experienced, physically and mentally, to be believed. It defied words, but no one who put their mind to it failed. Those who put their mind to it had a 100% success rate. I can't emphasize it enough – *those who put their mind to it did not fail, not once.*

Item 6: Never back down from a fat-fight. Never, ever give in when you start a fat-fight. Start it, but don't finish it. Never finish the fight. Keep fighting, because fat has no finish line. Fat won't give up. Fat won't give in. If you can do it alone, go in by yourself. If you can't do it alone, call for back-up, but never, ever back down. Don't listen to negative voices, especially the one inside your head, because you can work it out by shutting them out.

Item 7: This book is for anyone who wants to get in the best shape of their life and stay there. It explains how I beat the odds, changing countless minds, and allowing them to lose fat and get into their best shape. It contains the exact same message every one of the thousands I've coached and taught have heard. It contains the same tone, same body language, and the same direct blunt-force honesty. I don't pull punches. Winning the fat fight isn't for the meek. My system is called the *X Fitness System*. It teaches, in order of importance, what has worked in my life long fight versus fat, and what *has not* worked. It explains that fat-fighting is a series of continuous decisions that form either Fat Habits or Strong Habits. How to build will-power is more important than what to eat, and lift, and how much to run. My workout program and meal plan will be explained in the rest of the series. What I eat, lift, and how much I run is important, but it's secondary to will-power, self-discipline, and motivation. Meal plans and workout programs have zero value without *will-power*. No guts, big gut.

This is only book one of *Fat Losing*, which I'm calling: *Psychology of Fat Fighting*. There will be many books, a series, because of the *extent of content*. I tried to write just one book, but it's almost impossible, because the content would be the size of an encyclopedia. Fat losing is not quantum physics. I'll try to make the explanation as simple as possible. But the process is not simple. Dividing the content into a series of short books is the only way I know how to manage the whopping volume of material. You can decide how much you want to buy, if anything. After you've read book one, you can make the decision to continue buying more or stop. I don't want you to buy an over-sized textbook at an over-sized price and regret it after the first chapter.

Introduction

Here's what it feels like to be an obese, dysfunctional 12 year-old based on my experience:

1. *You dread taking off your shirt.* You dread summer. You dread phys-ed class. You dread little league sports. You dread facing the people who saw you without your shirt on.

2. *It takes a lot of guts.* Literally. My gut grew and grew, but nothing made a bigger impact than the day I saw bumps. My gut had bumps on it. Bumps of fat were all around my gut. Unsightly and unseemly bumps. Depending on perspective, we are blessed or cursed with long-term memory. The good news is the image of gut-bumps is stored in my memory, and the delete button is broke. The image has never failed to drive me in the gym, the kitchen, or on the treadmill. The bad news is that I kept seeing the image of gut-bumps long after they actually disappeared.

3. *You can't find clothes that fit.* No matter how you cut it, (excuse the pun) nothing fits right. The result is a *misfit*.

4. *A misfit is treated differently.* In my case, like a freak. It forced me to turn into another kind of freak.

5. *Inner hell.* My childhood obesity became an inner hell, because the potential of adolescent obesity stared me in the face. Then the potential of adult obesity turned up the temperature. Nothing happens until you reach a boiling point. It takes you to the *Crossroad*, where the most important exercise of all happens – the exercise of free will. The fire at the Crossroad either burns you up, or it fuels a drive that can't be stopped; a drive out of hell.

This list of five factors is the core of my fat-losing program. This list is my *motivation* and my *drive*. The list lit a fire, fuelling a *life-long* challenge. Not a 30-day challenge, nor a 60-day challenge, or even a 90-day challenge. It extended my playing career forever, with no retirement in sight. Without it, I would have quit long ago, because the fight would have been too hard, even though it's really over only one issue – growth. Fat cells don't disappear. Once you're fat, they never leave. They just shrink. Fat-fighting has one objective – stunt fat-cell growth. Don't let fat grow, because once it starts, it will grow out of control.

I've worked out continuously for 43 years in a 100% natural way. I have never taken steroids. I have never used performance enhancing drugs of any kind. I have never used any fat-burners or any illegal drugs of any kind. Why? For one reason: fear; several kinds of fear. It started with my parents – fear of the *horrible consequences* if they caught me. Bad stuff would have happened if I had come home wasted from drugs. It even made me stop drinking in my early 20's. Then my fear progressed from ey witness evidence. I saw the *side effects* of drugs. I've seen people wasted since high school, wasting their minds, wasting their bodies, and wasting their lives. It continued all the way through my police career. I saw people wasting time on the clock *being wasted*. Then, there was the fear of *hypocrisy*. I've told thousands of student-athletes the same message for decades, thousands of times: *steroid-use is a confession that you can't take it*. Taking steroids is an admission that you can't handle the natural struggle. Using drugs is hardcore evidence that you don't have what it takes. Steroids produce artificiality – artificial muscle, and artificial toughness. Steroids promote the great contradiction – synthetic toughness; artificial tough talk about artificially tough workouts. My Facebook news-feed is plastered with daily pro-wrestling style carnival-barking from the artificially-produced segment of the fitness industry. Steroid-aided workouts are not real. Steroid aided bodies are not real.

I've told my football teams over and over again that steroid users are not to be feared. Don't worry about lining up across from a steroid-user, because drug-induced performance is superficial. Steroid-users will crack under *4th-quarter pressure*. Every competition, every real-life situation, has the equivalent of 4th quarter pressure, where fatigue tries to shift the balance of power by draining it. The difference between winning and losing in any competition, in sports or real-life, is who can withstand 4th-quarter pressure better. The only one way to develop resistance to it is by beating the natural struggle. Steroid-users don't understand the experience or concept of the *natural struggle*. Those who by-pass the natural struggle via drugs will never fully develop the iron-will needed to endure 4th-quarter pressure. 4th-quarter pressure will crush them. That's the message I've communicated to student-athletes for decades. And it's worked out.

I *never* have and *never* will make ridiculous claims that you will lose X number of pounds in X number of weeks. Fat-losing doesn't follow a rigid, predictable scoreboard. You will score points, give up points, get ahead, or fall behind, but you will never predict with 100% certainty how much you will lose and win within a specific time clock. The chances of going undefeated against fat are next to none. Fat will fight to come back. Fat will fight dirty. Fat will never give up its fight. Fat will try to break you. Fat will try to make you give up. *Fat doesn't attack your gut first, it attacks your guts first – your mind.* Fat will attack your will. Fat will try to make you lose your guts before you lose your gut.

That's why fat-fighting starts at the top. Building your mind builds your body. That's also why fat-fighting doesn't have an off-season. One game leads to another. The true secret is to build a winning streak with a streak of fat losing. Fat losing doesn't just happen. Nothing just happens. This has a dual meaning: it doesn't happen automatically or overnight, and it doesn't happen by accident. Fat wins or fat loses by design, by the exercise of free will. Here's the key: change the focus. Change the *focus* of how you perceive fat fighting. Changing the *focus*, changes the *outcome*. If an obese, dysfunctional 12-year old can do it, so can you.

Chapter 1
Fat Habits: Losing the Battle of the Mind

∞

Fat-fighting is the only game where losing is winning. Losing fat for a while is not winning. It's a temporary victory, but not long-term winning. To win the fat fight, you have to lose more than fat. You have to lose the *fat habits* that keep making you lose the battle of the mind.

Winning the fat fight starts at the top and works down. It starts with mindset, a losing mentality that won't quit, especially when the fight reaches the toughest point – 4th quarter pressure. I've defined this as the *Crossroad*. It's a life-altering fork in the road, because it forces you to make a choice: break-down, or break-through. The break-point is guaranteed to happen during every fat-fight. The biggest challenge is the *double-team effect,* where your mind turns against you. Your mind will conjure up exaggerated mental fatigue in a feeble attempt to weaken your defenses so you'll give in and give up. If you don't win the mind games, it doesn't matter what nutrition program you try, workout program you try, or supplements you buy. The mind will lie to you, and then you'll quit.

Winning the mind game at the *Crossroad* is just the start of the fight; it's only a warm-up. Immediately following, you have to spill your guts to lose the gut. Sustained work, sustained exertion, and sustained effort are required. The secret is *continuity*, that is, conduct consistency. *Breaking* past the *break*-point is not enough. There has to be no *break* in the action.

Self-truth
The most over-looked and under-rated factor in losing fat is self-truth. The psychology of fat loss is a mind game that boils down to one issue – self-truth. Your physical shape is directly

connected to the extent of truth and lies that you tell yourself. Every human wages a non-stop inner war between truth and self-deception. We win some and we lose some. Where we end up depends on our win-loss record – how much self-truth we believe, or how much self-deception we believe. Breaking even won't break through the break-point. A .500 record isn't enough. A losing record definitely won't cause you to lose fat. Only a winning record will cut it. Cutting through the self deception cuts through the fat.

Therein lies the true secret to winning the battle of the mind: being honest with yourself. The difference between fitness success and failure is the extent of truth and lies that are tolerated and rewarded. Among all the athletes and students I've taught, the battle between self-honesty and self-dishonesty has always been the primary difference between their successes and failures.

Two Fat Habits

How you manage waste directly affects how you manage your *waist*. Fat Habits are waste mis-management that leads to *waist* mis-management. Waste mis-management is a ***junk collection*** that accumulates waste and expands the waist.

There are two Fat Habits that, left unchecked, will keep forcing you lose the battle of the mind, and stop you from losing fat. Both center on junk collection:

1. Junk that you consume – toxic waste products.

2. Junk that consumes your time – wasted time.

Junk that you consume is divided into two categories: solid and liquid.

Liquid junk includes the top two fat-builders – soft drinks and alcohol. *Soft drinks make you soft*; guaranteed. *Getting wasted expands your waist*; guaranteed. This is not scolding, or preaching, or sermonizing, or pontificating. It's simply the truth. I have told thousands of people I've coached that I personally don't give a shit what people do with their private lives. I really don't. But I do care when it affects the lives of others. Here are two examples of when I care about other people getting wasted: drunk drivers, and junk drivers.

I believe that drunk driving is attempted murder. Drunk drivers are potential killers. Getting wasted in the privacy of your own home is your decision, your choice, and your exercise of free will. So is your hangover and expanded waist. But getting behind the wheel of a car makes you a public enemy.

Junk drivers are teammates who drive with *junk hanging* over them when it's time to *show up and back-up*. The concept of showing-up and backing-up applies to every team sport or team profession I've been a part of. Survival depends on your team showing-up and backing-up. That means being *fully present*, not *hung-over* from being wasted the night before. You give up the right to be an asshole when your team depends on you. You forfeit the right to be soft when your teammates' lives and health are on the line. So if you don't want to show-up and back-up for yourself, do it for your team; your professional team and your personal team. Don't forget that your family is a teamtoo. Your family is the most important team, the one that looks up to you. Your family needs you to show-up and back-up.

Own up to it. Soft drink and alcohol abusers will try to blame the coach, the workout program, the gym, the spouse, or anyone else they can point a finger to except for themselves. Don't blame a workout program if you binge drink on the side. Don't blame your personal trainer if you absorb alcohol and soft drinks like a sponge. Don't blame your gym, or its equipment, or its floor design...Blame yourself. There are two magic words that are guaranteed to change your life: *MY FAULT.* Taking personal responsibility is life-altering. It's the first step toward lasting positive change. The moment you start blaming yourself, you have identified the true problem: Your lack of will-power, your lack of self discipline, your lack of drive, and your lack of motivation.

Junk solid food is the next category of consumable junk. A complete list of junk solid food does not need to be detailed in an e-book. I won't waste your time with hundreds of pages listing all the junk solid food that you already know about. To prevent waste, I'll give you *my* definition of junk solid food, and one that I live by: Anything other than un-fried fish or chicken, egg whites, brown rice, and any fruit or vegetable. That's it. Anything else is the equivalent of poison to my system. When I stick to these, I feel alive with a flat stomach. It's that simple. My list of non-junk liquid is even shorter:

1. 3 litres (minimum) a day of Muscle Water, my own muscle-recovery concoction that I started drinking years ago. It's been life-altering, and has brought my workout to higher levels.

2. Caffeinated coffee (first half of the day).

3. Decaf coffee (second half of the day).

That's it. I drink no other substance. My workouts are getting better and better with age.

Junk that consumes your time is the second Fat Habit. It represents another waste; wasted time. The dreaded fat-builder: *inactivity.* Idling. Stuck in neutral, or worse, stuck in park. I activity is an anabolic agent of fat that eventually leads to inner conflict, the result of being in the shape you don't want to be in. A sedentary life leads to inner strife. Inactivity will pack on weight at warp-speed. Physical exertion will unpack it. I have warned everyone I've coached to *never* retire from physical activity when their playing days are over. Don't fall into the trap of retiring from physical activity before your 21st birthday. My definition of "playing days" is different than the conventional definition. "Playing days" is not reserved for organized sports. "Playing days" go beyond the organized sports career. "Playing days" includes the natural physical activity engaged in by children and adolescents, hours of playing *outside;* working at manual labor something that was possible before the Screen Age arrived. The Age that caused Screen Paralysis, that is, an era of zombies stuck to the screens of their cell phones, laptops, video games, TVs, and every other next-gen addictive gadget. I've warned young people to extend their "playing career" to forever by never retiring. Keep moving. Don't let the fire burn out.

The best way to keep the fire going is a commitment to burn calories instead of counting them. Rather than being consumed with the calorie balance-sheet or focusing on calorie consumption, upset the balance by changing the focus to burning more and more calories. Build an inner fire, and burn more calories than you're used to burning. Raise the heat instead of measuring every ounce of what you eat. Build a calorie imbalance through motion. Movement burns calories. Physical activity burns more. Extreme physical exertion burns even more.

The conventional way of counting calories involves the obsession of reducing calorie-consumption to meet the anemic number of calories burned by a person with a sedentary, inactive life. Focusing on *calorie-consumption reduction* often leads to frustration, because it's the *wrong* focus. It leaves you in the worst shape possible; hungry and weak. You're defenseless. You can't win the fat fight by constantly lowering the calorie bar or dropping calories to meet the idling-rate of calorie-burning. Doing so is the equivalent of running on empty. Your body is a high-performance machine. Fuel it instead of fooling it. Fuel your body with premium grade instead of fooling it with the spoils. High-grade equals high octane; low-grade is equal to low-gain.

Instead of trying to run on empty and idle, fill the tank and drive. Changing the focus changes the outcome. Make calorie-burning your top priority, and match calorie-consumption accordingly. You'll change your physical and mental shape by burning more calories instead of calorie-deprivation. Make a commitment to build an inner fire, and burn as many calories as possible *every* day. Then, reduce junk calories. Change the focus to burning more calories and matching quality calories to fuel an active lifestyle, not vice-versa. Don't try to fuel an inactive life that's stuck in park. Conserving fuel will not save your physical and mental environment. The focus of consuming fewer calories than you burn is the wrong focus. It softens you. What you focus on can only grow. Focus on calorie-burning and calorie-burning will grow.

Focusing on calorie-intake over calorie-burning is inside-the-box thinking. Think outside the box until the box disappears altogether. Focus on *raising the temperature* daily with a Calorie Burning Program that increases calories burned because of increased physical exertion. Make a commitment to reach the *boiling point,* the degree of physical work that strikes the *mismatch*, the calorie-imbalance where you burn more than you consume, and do it without counting.

Calorie-Burning 101, an introductory 3-step Calorie-burning Program

1. Lift The Screen. Reduce screen time to the bare essential. The determining factor that calculates essential screen time is a simple 4-word question: "Is there a return?" Essential Screen time is an investment that guarantees

a return; financially or intellectually. Essential screen time improves quality of life. Non-essential screen time is clock-killing; a waste of time. Non-essential screen time promotes seclusion and isolation leading to idling, a sedentary inactive life that regresses shape and progresses fat build-up. Replace non essential screen time with any kind of movement. Push away from non-essential screen involvement. Lifting the Screen opens your eyes to real-life possibilities and opportunities.

2. Carry weight other than excessive bodyweight. Weight is a paradox, and so is carrying weight. Weight can soften or strengthen depending on whether you carry it around your waist, or carry it to exercise. Carrying excessive bodyweight weakens. Carrying external weight strengthens. Be creative. Take every opportunity to pick up some weight, lift it, and carry it. Lifting and carrying the right weight is miraculous. It transforms your body and mind.

3. Manual labor works off more fat than working out. I was blessed to experience back-breaking manual labor in a flour mill as my high school job. I strongly recommend any kind of manual labour either for a living, or as a supplement to a desk job. Manual labour solves all your calorie-counting problems. Here are five reasons why I wasblessed to have experienced extreme manual labour:

    1. *Carrying heavy weight removed heavy weight.* Carrying 140 lb. flour bags 8 hours a day transformed my body and mind. In addition to my weight-training program, extreme manual labour transformed my childhood physical and mental obesity. Extreme manual labour was a solution to my biggest adolescent problems.

2. *Diet solution.* The power of extreme physical exertion removed the anxiety of calorie-counting, and all the other time-wasting nonsense associated with dieting. I ate to fuel the next work day. I worked with the strongest adults I have ever met in my life. The strongest physically, mentally, and emotionally. I never saw any of them dieting. I never heard anyone mention the words *calories* or *carbs*. In fact, I never heard complaining, whining, or excuse-making. I learned the power of S.U.A.L. - **S**hut **U**p **A**nd **L**ift. A diet of hard labour is the solution.

3. *Gratitude.* I have deeply appreciated my professions that I worked in. Policing, teaching, coaching, writing, and business all have extreme challenges, but none called out every fiber of physical and mental strength the way 8 hours of continuous lifting did.

4. *Re-wiring.* Hard labour eliminated Fat Habits, and replaced them with Strong Habits. If you're looking for a true mental and physical makeover, go work in a factory.

5. *Soul-lifting.* I learned the spiritual connection between physical strength and inner peace. Extreme physical work is the ultimate body and mind detoxifier. It purifies the soul. It was my first and only experience with a poison-free work environment. The bad news is that I never experienced it again in any other occupation. The good news is it taught me how to build a team. I build a team through extreme work in the gym and on the field. It's never failed to work out.

Chapter 1 Summary

- Changing Fat Habits is the true solution to being in shape.

- Starts by cleaning up the junk in your life.

- Make a list of all junk food that you consume. Commit to eliminating all of it from your life. Changing junk food and junk time is the primary solution to fat losing.

- Make a list of all junk that wastes your time and makes you sedentary. Change gears. Move from park to drive.

Chapter 2
Psych101: Winning the Battle of the Mind

∞

"Football-practice mentality is one of the true secrets to high-performance in any sport, any profession, any business. It's the difference between winning and losing. Football-practice mindset is life-altering. Builds lasting change. The reason is what it's made of. There's a secret formula to it that transforms. But the formula is not obvious. It starts as a mystery but it's easily solved. Those who have experienced it, never forget it because the change is permanent. The good news is that the football field is not the only place to experience it. The bad news is you don't know what you're missing until you try it."

Code of Conduct, SWAT Football series, Gino Arcaro

The biggest challenge I've had is teaching student-athletes how to work extremely hard physically *and* mentally to survive in high-risk activity. The majority of rookies I've coached and taught are out-of-shape, physically and mentally. That means they are prone to *underachieving*; achieving under their potential. Not fully using their natural gifts. Underachieving is not created equal. There are soft cases and hardcore cases, but all underachieving leads to higher *body fat* and *mind fat* percentage; they are directly connected. A soft mind leads to a soft body. There's no escaping it. The body only does what the mind tells it to do, and it doesn't do what it's not told to do.

Science now has given us evidence of what has always been suspected: the mind quits long before the body does.

The mind is a quitter by human nature.[2] For the first time, science proved that activating muscle-power depends on will-power and

---

2   University of Zurich (2011, December 5). How muscle fatigue originates in the head. ScienceDaily. Retrieved February 11, 2012, from http://www.sciencedaily.com / releases/2011/12/111205081643.htm

inner motivation, because the mind sends a false-alarm intended to kill will. The mind is soft by nature, a coddling enabler, hell-bent on making life easy. Translation: don't over-exert, don't break limits, don't reach new levels, and stay confined inside the safety of the smallest boxes possible. The mind is prone to work-aversion. It doesn't like to leave its comfort zone, and it will play expert mind games to get you to give in and give up. The secret weapon the mind uses is lies; deception. It sends false signals trying to trick you into giving up before the job is done.[3] Having a football-practice mentality is a strong defense against mind games.

Strong Habits

Football-practice mentality blasts away every Fat Habit, replacing them with Strong Habits. The difference between Strong Habits and Fat Habits is *right from wrong*. I define a Strong Habit simply as the *right* thing to *do* and *doing* it *right*. Three separate concepts emerge from that definition. The *right* thing to *do* is the *right* call to make; the right strategy or tactic. Actually *doing it* means having the drive to put it in motion; the will to make it happen. *Doing it right* means flawless execution. Therefore, a Strong Habit has three parts: make the right call, put it in motion, and execute flawlessly. Flawless knowledge, flawless will, and flawless execution.

Never underestimate the power of a *Strong Habit*. It is the solution to every problem known to wo/mankind, including Fat Losing. Not knowing the right thing to do exposes habits to guesswork and randomness. Knowing the right thing to do will put you on the right track but, by itself, it will never guarantee success. Knowing what to do is only the starting point. Intentions remain dreams until they are driven into action. The drive will crash unless the right directions are taken. You'll be lost. The main cause of failure is being *lost*.

---

3   Ibid.

"Lost" is a state of mind; a cognitive path that's headed the *wrong* way. The wrong direction never leads you to what you're looking for. One or any combination of all three flaws makes you lost – flawed knowledge, flawed will, or flawed execution. Being lost results in losing except when it comes to fat. Fat scores points when you're lost.

Every achievement, including being in shape, has a pathway of Strong Habits. Every accomplishment is made up of building blocks; the right things to do and the will to consistently do them right. Strong Habits are not the mystery they appear to be. The right things are actually common sense. It doesn't take a scientist to know that beer, pizza, and grease-dripping wings will make you fat. You don't need to be a nutritional expert to know the right foods from wrong foods. You don't need a graduate degree to know that inactivity won't ever get you in the best shape of your life. But common sense gets lost, becoming a victim of mind games. Self-deception leads to full-blown delusion, which is a total departure from reality, that is, lost. The only solution is *overcoming self.* Defeat your worst enemy: yourself and your mind.

Self-overcoming

Every athlete I've coached who was out-of-shape or failed to get in shape did so because they *chose* it, exercising their free will. Those who got in the best shape of their lives did so because they *chose* it, also exercising their free will. Both types of exercise are directly connected to overcoming self – one does, and one doesn't. One type of free-will exercise breaks your will. The other type of free will exercise builds your will. It builds an iron-will. The difference between fat losing and fat gaining is iron-will. No one is born with iron-will. Iron-will doesn't just happen. It doesn't happen automatically. It doesn't happen overnight. It doesn't happen at random. It doesn't happen by accident. Iron-will happens for a reason. Iron-will is developed through Strong Habits. It's built by conscious decisions that turn into work. Iron-will is shaped in the mind. Then it shapes your body.

Here are the basics that build Strong Habits of fat losing that turn into iron-will. This is the guts of Psychology 101; a waste management program that manages your waist:

1. *Become fearless of the investment.* Changing your attitude toward the *investment*, changes the outcome. Remove the *presumption* of pain. All success, including fitness success, requires an investment. Getting in the best shape of your life takes *investment capital*, the investment of five properties: physical, intellectual, emotional, spiritual, and financial. Every investment has a high price-tag. Fear of making the investment leads to failing to lose fat and failing to get in the best shape of your life. Paying the full price follows the 90-10 Rule: 90% of people are not willing to pay full price; 10% are. However, 100% are capable. It's not a 50-50 split. The reason is too painful to explain. It's the *presumption* of pain. There's a common presumption that investing in fat-losing or fitness success of any kind is painful. The presumption of pain a most automatically accompanies the thought of investment. The reason is poor conditioning; brainwashing. The presumption of pain is one of a long list of conventional myths that people have been conditioned to believe. It starts with the common attitude toward *struggle*. All success, including fitness success, requires a natural struggle that, by nature, is not comfortable. Most view the *natural struggle* as painful. The natural struggle is a Darwinism process that cuts 90%, those with a low threshold of pain brought on by the unwillingness to endure discomfort. Low

pain-tolerance is in the mind. It's the outcome of prior mind games won by the mind. Change your perspective of the struggle, and your outcome will change. Change your mindset toward the investment, and your outcome will change.

2. *Focus on the investment reward, not the investment consequence.* Nothing changes until you see rewards instead of consequences. The secret is to change your mind; change your perspective of the struggle so you focus on the reward. Two steps will change the focus: Step 1: *Change your language* – replace *struggle* with *process*. Step 2: Focus on the reward by shifting the spotlight onto 3 benefits: (i) Health (ii) Feeling (iii) Challenge. Good health is the greatest blessing in life. No material possession will ever replace good health. The inner peace of being in shape outweighs the inner hell of being out-of-shape. To get through the daily grind, focus on the miracle of the *pump* that the process gives you; the physical, intellectual, emotional, and spiritual *rush* that is guaranteed through exertion. Challenges are powerful motivators. They counter-act one of the evils that plague routine daily life: boredom. The reward of being in the very best shape possible is a powerful remedy to the negative side-effects of being bored out of your mind. Health. Feeling. Challenge. What you focus on grows. Change the focus, and change the outcome.

3. *Change the presumption of imagined consequences to the presumption of real consequences by thinking of the alternative.* Anything that is hard to do triggers the *presumption* of imagined, bad consequences including, but not limited to, pain, discomfort, and failure. The presumption of imagined consequences is a powerful blocker that will

stop you before and even after you get started. Falling victim to this mind game will prevent you from even trying. The secret is to change your perspective from *imagined consequences to real consequences* by thinking of the alternative to not getting in shape. The alternative is a life sentence of being unhealthy as a fat and overweight individual. If you want something bad enough, you have to not want something else even more. According to the Law of Survival, something has to be done to not let the actual worst consequence happen. If you don't take drastic action in the face of the threat of the *real* worst consequence, the worst will happen. If you want to get in the very best shape, you have to not want to be in the very worst shape. The quickest way to change your focus is fear. Be intensely afraid of fat. Fear the pain of being overweight. When the pain of being overweight outweighs the pain of losing weight, fat losing will ha pen. When you get weak and want to quit, think of the alternative. Think of the real consequences of being overweight and out-of-shape for the *rest of your life.*

4. *Make fat losing a basic survival need.* There's a common motivational cliché overused by coaches during pre-game speeches and halftime speeches: "WHOEVER WANTS IT THE MOST, WINS." I disagree. Everyone *wants* to win, but not everyone *needs* to win. No one *wants* to lose. No one *wants* to fail. Yet, not everyone wants to pay the price to win. Not everyone wants to make the investment to succeed, usually because of the cost. The difference between succeeding and failing at something extremely hard to do is *need.* Those who *need* to win won't accept losing. The same applies to fat losing. Those who *need* it, lose fat. But needs are not created equal. The most powerful need is a *basic survival need.* When the

need to be in-shape becomes the same as breathing and eating, you will stay in-shape for life. You will win the battle of your mind, because basic survival needs beat out the mind's false signals to quit every single time. Basic survival needs are the most powerful motivators. You will fight to fill them.

5. *Find a compelling need that forces a self-generated performance demand.* There are two challenges to making fat loss a basic survival need:

    a. There's limited room for additional basic survival needs, there's just enough space for the essential ones. Making more room takes work.

    b. A progression is needed for an ordinary need to become a basic survival need.

The key is a *use of force* tactic. It's an inner motivation that forces the mind to make a self-generated performance demand, the science of conditioning the mind to make only one choice by removing all other alternatives. A *performance demand* is not a request, it's an order. It removes discretion. Only one decision is available – no others, no alternatives, no escape. Performance demands can originate externally or internally. The highest level of performance demand, but toughest level to achieve, is the internal kind; the self-generated performance demand. It's the true secret to sustained performance. When you reach that stage, fat losing becomes internalized and hardwired. You won't fail, because you won't accept any other choice. No other alternatives will exist. A self-generated performance demand is hardcore iron will. It's the strongest inner drive attainable. The ability to make self-generated performance demands is the top-level of self-reliance. It's an independence from external motivators. The ability to make self-generated performance demands is the only foolproof way to keep your soul on fire for good. No one is born with the ability to make self-generated performance demands. The skill is built and developed over time by a progression of stronger compelling needs. Soul-searching and brutal self-honesty are the driving forces that uncover your compelling needs. They form your inner motivation to something that grows in intensity. An inner fire that gets bigger and stronger. My inner motivation for fat losing has gone through 5 phases of compelling needs:

- Phase 1: Started working out at age 12 to fight fat and the negative effects of a dysfunctional childhood.

- Phase 2: Worked out heavier to compete in little league football and high school football.

- Phase 3: Worked out even heavier for street survival during policing career.

- Phase 4: Intensity heightened when my strength-coaching career started, trying to keep up with the athletes I coached in the gym. Being a role model for my team wasn't enough. As the head coach, I had to be the strongest pound-for-pound athlete on the team.

- Phase 5: Intensity climbed to its highest level to fight the clock. I will not cave into age. 55 is only a number. My workouts are more intense today than 30 years ago, and I'm in the best shape of my life.

Build your own list of inner motivation with levels of compelling needs that will make the *biggest impact in your life*. The key is impact. The secret to identifying what will make the biggest impact is to *find your greatest fears*. What scares you the most is a problem that can be solved by developing a compelling need.

Appeal to your conscience

This is the most powerful way to becoming an expert at making self-generated performance demands. This is the true secret to building the iron-will needed for life-long fat losing. Appealing to the conscience is the most underrated, most ignored factor in fat losing and getting in shape. I believe the reason why it's the most ignored is because it's not sexy, or glamorous, and there's no magic pill for it. But it works. Appealing to the conscience skyrockets performance, including getting in shape.

The purpose of appealing to your conscience is to *make the conscience work*. Triple meaning: make it work out, make it work right, and make it do all the work. Nothing is more important for any kind of performance, including fat losing and life-long fitness. Appealing to your own conscience guarantees that you will do exactly what it takes to keep you fit. A strong conscience will instinctively choose right from wrong. Therein lies the key: consistently deciding right over wrong develops Strong Habits. When the conscience knows right from wrong with 100% certainty, you will make the conscience work out, you will make the conscience work right, and you will make the conscience do all the work.

Making the conscience work out means to strengthen it through positive reps; referring to right-from-wrong training, that is, making consistent decisions that choose the right thing to do over the wrong. A strong conscience is your strongest advantage in your fight against fat. No force is stronger. A strong conscience will force you to do all the right things to lose weight and get in the very best shape of your life. No one is born with a strong conscience, however. It's built. It's developed over time through reps. A well built conscience does what no other force of nature can do. It flips a natural, inner switch that is your Compulsion to Do Right.[4] This theoretical concept is *my* extension of Theodore Reik's theory of the *Compulsion to Confess*. Reik, a Freudian

---

4   Tribute to a Masterpiece. The Compulsion to Confess by Theodore Reik.(1959) Grove Press, New York. Reik, a Freudian psychiatrist, pioneered the theory of the compulsion to confess, theorized that all humans have a compulsion to confess, an inner need to tell the truth. I've extended the theory by adding the Compulsion to Do Right.

psychiatrist, theorized that all humans have a compulsion to confess, an inner need to tell the truth. The compulsion to confess is an urge that we all have to solve inner conflicts caused by guilt of doing wrong. It's the conscience's way of reaching inner peace by resolving our inner conflicts by telling the truth. In other words, we need to spill our guts. I extended the theory by adding the Compulsion to Do Right, adding a physical component to the theory. It's an inner urge to *do* the right thing when we believe it's the right thing to do. The conscience will work like hell to get us to do what's right *if* we believe it's the right thing to do.

The decision to get in shape is the conscience's way of resolving the inner conflict of being overweight and out-of-shape by forcing us *to do the right physical things needed to get in shape.* Our Compulsion to Do Right is the conscience's way of lifting the crushing weight off our shoulders *only after* we believe it's wrong to have let ourselves get out-of-shape. The conscience will do all the work for us by forcing us to eat right and exercise *if* we *believe* it's wrong for us to be overweight and out-of shape. Our beliefs are the starting point for the Compulsion to Do Right to work its magic. We have to strongly believe that being in-shape is the right thing. We have to believe it is our responsibility to maximize our health. We have to believe that it's wrong to have let ourselves go. We have to sincerely believe that being in good shape matters, that it's relevant and significant in our lives. We have to believe that being in the very best shape has a distinct life purpose. When the right beliefs about fitness are solidly entrenched, the conscience won't allow us to get away with doing wrong. We'll pay a price that will force us to change back to our beliefs. When our conscience works, we work out. When our conscience is strong, we get strong. But the opposite also applies. If we don't have hardcore beliefs about fitness and being in-shape, then not being in shape won't matter. It won't trigger the inner compulsion to do what's right, and you'll quit trying. Soft conscience is equal to soft body. A strong conscience doesn't just force us to do what is socially right – stop u committing heinous crimes against society – it also stops u committing crimes against self.

Cognitive dissonance

When we contradict ourselves by acting contrary to our beliefs, we pay for it. We suffer an inner conflict called *cognitive dissonance,*[5] an inner hell of guilt intended to cause us to change our ways. That's the good news; it's a hell of a motivator. Cognitive dissonance can create a powerful incentive that drives us to make positive change by deciding to do what's right, and to fix what we don't like about ourselves. Doing the right thing eliminates cognitive dissonance for good. It's the long-term solution that casts out the inner demons that feed the specific problem that invited them in in the first place. Doing the right thing brings inner peace. In the case of fitness, getting in shape brings the inner peace that we all desire and cherish. The bad news is that the same cognitive dissonance can be abated by a temporary solution called *rationalization.* Rationalization is our inner bullshit system, the one that make excuses to justify why we're in the bad shape we're in. Rationalization can be full of lies, alibis, and denials.

Here's the best example of rationalization: genetics. Heredity. I'm guilty of it. I have blamed my parents on those cloudy days when my abs disappeared. "My mother was obese her entire life. Over 90 years." The climate is another example. I blame the cold, snow, and lack of sun. Occasionally, I still use these pathetic forms of self-pity to bullshit myself. It makes me feel better after I over eat and fill up with greasy fries and pizza dripping

---

5   Tribute to a masterpiece. A theory of cognitive dissonance by Leon Festinger (1957) Evanston, IL: Row, Peterson. Leon Festinger pioneered the concept of cognitive dissonance in 1957. Cognitive dissonance is mental conflict brought on by acting in contradiction to personal beliefs. Cognitive dissonance is both a motivator and a change agent. It compels a change – change the belief or change the act.

with enough oil to top off my car engine – for about a minute. But I've learned to control it. I beat it every time. I've learned the secret to stop rationalizing and do what's right. I don't take

any time off from working out. Never have, never will. No sick days, no vacation days, no weekends off, no statutory holidays off, and no summers off. I have a Spartan nutrition plan, minus a few moments of weakness. All because I learned the secret: change my mindset toward doing the right things from being painful to pleasurable. Getting in top shape happens only after your look forward to eating right and exercising right instead of dreading it. You won't get in top shape if you believe its hell to eat right and exercise right.

Dread the wrong things. Make the wrong things too much to handle. Fear waste. There won't be any long-term change until you fear consuming waste and fear inactivity. Lasting change happens only when being out-of-shape scares you, and when rationalizing your Fat Habits terrifies you. Until then, nothing will work out.

Cognitive dissonance forces us to change for the better, or stay the same and get worse. Cognitive dissonance forces us to exercise free will. Make the call. Either start doing the right thing, or justify wrong with rationalized fiction. Left to our own devices, we won't always choose the right thing to do. Similar to a multiple-choice test, too many selections tempt us to guess. Or cheat. Or even leave it blank. I've learned the secret of beating the temptation to habitually rationalize. Chronic rationalization starts a chain reaction that lights the wrong type of inner fire: true inner hell. Chronic rationalization leads to delusion, which leads to mind fat, which leads to body fat, which leads to regrets, which leads to resentment, which leads to the worst hell of all – bitterness. The only choice is to stop rationalizing. But that's easier said than done.

Chapter 2 Summary

- Changing your mindset changes your mind games.

- No meal plan, no workout plan, no diet will work out unless you win the battle of the mind by appealing to your conscience to do its work so you can do yours.

- If being in bad shape doesn't bother your conscience, you won't bother to change. Guaranteed.

- If being in bad shape *does* bother your conscience, you will change. Guaranteed.

- How much your conscience bothers you about the shape you're in determines the strength of your self-generated performance demands.

Chapter 3
The Turnaround

F'd up

Appealing to your conscience is the most powerful way to make self-generated performance demands, the type that make lasting life-changes. Appealing to your conscience is the true secret of making the turnaround, the life-altering transformation that will get you in top shape and keep you there. But appealing to your conscience is easier said than done.

Everyone is capable of high-performance. Everyone is capable of making a *turnaround*. You can make a comeback from whatever shape you're in. I've seen the "Power of the Underdog." Over and over again, I've witnessed lost causes reach higher and higher by going deeper and deeper. The reason each time was pain; they had had enough of it. They were Fed-up with feeling F'd-up. It's a feeling that doesn't just happen. Nothing just happens. It's worked out by a strong conscience.

F'd up is fat caused by fitness flaws and failings. The most powerful change agent is pain. That's the *boiling point* that either sets your soul on fire to change for the better, or burns you up in an inner hell of unresolved conflict where you settle for getting worse. There are two types of pain that motivate:

1. Physical discomfort of being out-of-shape, of not being able to fit in clothes, or not being able to enjoy simple physical exertion without gasping for air.

2. Psychological discomfort of unde achieving, of not reaching your full potential; the pain of letting life slide by without fully experiencing what you want to experience.

Nothing changes until you cross the threshold that separates handling the pain and not tolerating it. The boiling point. You have to reach a temperature of inner hell to motivate you to make drastic change. The most powerful lasting change is any escape from hell. When something frees us from an inner hell, we're hooked. Escaping from hell needs a flawless plan, flawless execution, and most importantly, a flawless drive. The most fuel that drives you to accept nothing less than flawless execution is being Fed-up with being F'd-up. The point where you no longer can tolerate the wrong that you're doing to yourself. Reaching the boiling point doesn't just happen. Nothing just happens. You have to work at getting there. Either you get there on your own or you get there with back-up. In most cases, getting Fed-up with being F'd-up takes a team effort. Turnarounds don't happen on your own, or on their own, they have to be worked out.

I reached that point as an obese, dysfunctional 12-year old. I'd had enough. I was Fed-up with being F'd-up. I had reached the boiling point. Two options were available, but I canceled out the "getting worse" option. That left only one choice, which was a no brainer: Get better. Do the right things to get in shape. I put my mind to it and gave myself no escape. I made my first self-generated performance demand at the age of 12. It worked out. I learned to make another one, and another one, until making self-generated performance demands became automatic. The demands became second-nature; a force of nature hardwired through hardcore REPS – repeated exertion produces strength. Physically and mentally.

REPS are life-changers
High-quality and high-quantity REPS are life-altering. They're the *true secret* to making lasting change. A high volume of quality REPS is guaranteed to change your mind and body. High quality REPS are made up of doing the right things that lead to being

in top shape and *not doing* the wrong things that lead to bad shape. Positive REPS include:

- increasing physical-exertion time
- decreasing idling time
- increasing good food consumption
- decreasing bad food consumption

All reduction of waste is a positive REP. Every time you decline junk drinks and junk foods, you have executed a positive rep. Every time you decline to recline, you have executed a positive REP. Addition by subtraction. Removing waste counts. Removing waste adds up. Then, adding the right exercise and right food builds up. *Positive REPS add up and build up.* Positive REPs cut down mind fat. Body fat follows. The top-to-bottom chain reaction; mind fat reduction reduces body fat.

After I learned the secret, I coached it. I believe there is always a reason for hardship and adversity. One such reason is to learn how to solve a problem, and then share the solution. Coaching and teaching taught me that I wasn't alone. I wasn't the only one who was lost. In my opinion, I've coached more people who were lost than those who weren't. I realized that high body-fat doesn't always manifest in obesity. Sometimes, the revelation is frailty.

David vs. Goliath
I've coached and taught many frail people. I have never coached elite athletes at prestigious universities, high schools, or on professional teams. I've only coached and taught the *open-admission* athletes, those who couldn't fit into the higher standards of higher places. I've taught community college students, not Ivy-leaguers. I've coached at public schools, not Goliath-sized Catholic schools (*note*: I'm Catholic. This isn't Catholic-bashing, but there's nothing better than helping poor public school teams beat rich Catholic school teams).

There's no greater reward than knocking out Goliath. There's no stronger evidence that justifies extreme exertion than the little guy beating the big guy. It just doesn't get any better than that. It's the biggest life-changer a lost-cause student-athlete can experience, because it validates the highest REPSS of all: **R**ewarding **E**xertion **P**roduces **S**trength & **S**uccess.

I have witnessed countless open-admission lost-causes reduce their mind-fat and body-fat. There have been too many to count. It proves to me that anyone can do it. I did it, and they did it. None of us were anything special. None of us were genetically gifted. All of us had fitness flaws and failings of one kind or another. All of us faced big odds. And all of us beat the odds. We did it when we lowered our pain tolerance for being F'd-up.

Staying F'd up can hurt or not hurt. Both staying out-of-shape *and* getting in shape can be painful or pain-relieving. Eating right can be painful or painless…So can eating wrong. Exercising can be painful or pleasurable…So can idling. The one who hurts the most, loses. The one who hurts the least, wins. What is painful gets stopped. What is painless continues. We will fight like hell for what is pleasurable, and fight like hell to avoid what isn't.

When you make a conscious decision to classify Fat Habits as being brutally wrong, your own conscience will take over, and it will direct you to do the right things. *The direction of a strong conscience is the most underrated and most ignored factor in getting in top shape.* However, if eating right and exercising right fail to work out, it only proves that the conscience wasn't strong enough to do its job. Believing anything else is futile. Search your conscience when things go wrong, and you are guaranteed to discover the weakness, if you open your mind to it.

The Power of X

How do you appeal to your own conscience? How does a turn-around happen? How do you make lasting change? How do you make life-altering decisions that change the shape you're in? How do you solve fitness and fat problems? The solution is the *"Power of X."*

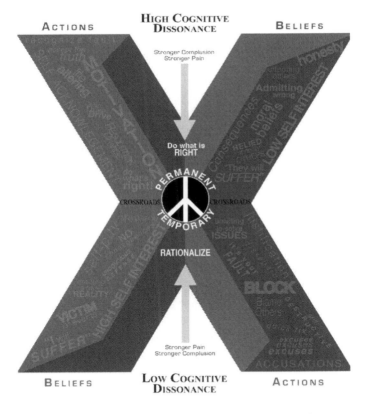

There is a driving force that causes your life to change when you make a "self-generated performance demand". The force relies on one fundamental principle: *make the conscience work to do what's right.* Triple meaning: Make it work out, make it work right, and make it do all the work. Strengthen the conscience by conditioning it to know exactly what the right things to do are. Use the conscience's strength to execute flawlessly, and let it do all the heavy lifting.

The Power of X illustrates that driving force is a *system* that *naturally* reveals and accepts the truth. The truth is synonymous with doing the right things to become what you need to be. The truth has to be accepted before it becomes lasting so that positive physical change can be made. The biggest barrier to change is taking the easy way out, that is, rationalizing and rejecting the truth, such as inventing a false reality… and then accepting it as being real.

"Truth" and "doing right" are natural psychological outcomes. Humans have a natural inner compulsion to tell the truth and do what's right. This compulsion is fueled by a need for inner peace and a feeling of guilt-free inner harmony achieved when actions align with moral beliefs.

The X has two primary features:

1. Two Gaps:

    a. The top half of the X is the upright V-shape. The space defined by the upright V has an informal name, and a formal name. The formal name is *"high cognitive dissonance gap."* The simplified, informal name is "V-Gap."

    b. The lower half of the X, the inverted V-shape is formally called, *"low cognitive dissonance gap"* or "A-Gap."

2. The Crossroad; the middle of the X represents inner peace.

Gap DNA
V-Gap and A-Gap share almost identical DNA. They represent the inner hell of "cognitive dissonance," defined as, "the conflict one feels by acting contrary to one's personal beliefs; guilt

caused by acknowledged wrongdoing." Cognitive dissonance is relieved by either admitting the wrong, or justifying it. *The only difference between V-Gap and A-Gap is the focus of the consequences of the wrong and the suffering caused.* The only way to resolve and relieve either gap cognitive dissonance is to close the gap. "Closing the gap" means making actions and beliefs cross paths. When actions and beliefs cross paths at the Crossroad in the middle of the X, the offender feels guilt-free, inner peace, balance, and harmony.

V-Gap guilt focuses on low self-interest. In other words, you believe someone else is suffering the worst consequence of you being out-of-shape. The cognitive dissonance that results is due to the "wrong" of being out-of-shape, that is, the relevance of being out-of-shape. The strongest relevance is the harm it's causing to others who are relying on you now, and to those who will be relying on you in the future. Every human being is, or will be, relied on by someone. The relevance of being in top shape starts with acknowledging the harm of being in bad shape and the connection it has to the potential harm to others.

A-Gap guilt focuses on high self-interest. You believe you are suffering the worst consequence of being out-of-shape. The resulting cognitive dissonance causes you justify your situation by rationalizing that there are no consequences, either to you or anyone else, and that it's not your fault. Permanent change won't happen because the right things are not acknowledged, accepted, and most importantly, not followed.

Reality
The *power* of the "X" is that it illustrates reality.

If you are overweight and out-of-shape, the truth of the situation is that you are operating in the bottom of the X (in the A-Gap), an area filled with self-destructive potential brought on by being unwilling or allegedly unable to solve a pressing problem. You are immersed in the worst mindset possible, one that is guaranteed to block all efforts to make positive change, i.e. excuse-making. You blame everyone and everything, except yourself, for being out-of-shape. This rationalization, the result of low cognitive dissonance, closes the Gap and allows you to reach the Cros road. In other words, if you don't feel badly about your situation, you've done an incredible job of rationalizing it. You experience a sense of peace in justifying your actions by blaming others. But the inner peace is only temporary; you'll sink back into the ever-widening, psychologically-chaotic A-Gap as self-pity and bullshit rear their ugly heads and force you to decide again: be truthful, or rationalize the wrong.

The goal is to close the A-Gap permanently by not only operating in the V-Gap, but by opening it as wide as possible; the wider the better. There is *only one way* to open the V-Gap: By *acknowledging* and *accepting the truth*. Honesty is the key. We are built to change what we don't like, but we have to not like it first and acknowledge that it is wrong. By being truthful, the V-Gap opens and does what it's supposed to do, which is activate high cognitive dissonance, triggering the inner compulsion to do what's right. As you are compelled and propelled toward the Crossroad, the Gap closes for good. True confession is permanent in relation to that wrongdoing. The guilt about that sin is erased.

Without high cognitive dissonance, you will never have the inner motivation and drive to make life-altering changes necessary. Without high cognitive dissonance, you will never push yourself to go through the true struggle of losing weight to get in shape. Without high cognitive dissonance, nothing will work out; not a meal plan, not an exercise program, and you'll even stop taking all the fat-burning supplements that you've spent a fortune on. If you want to change, high cognitive dissonance is a must, not an option. It starts with the truth.

Chapter 3 Summary

- When you are fed up with being F'd up, it's because you have reached the boiling point – inner hell.

- You have choice to operate in the A-gap or the V-gap and close it.

- Closing either gap will move you toward the Crossroad.

- One path to the middle of the "X" is to accept the truth by admitting that what you've been doing is wrong and it is not working out. Reaching the Crossroad on this path is the result of high cognitive dissonance. The feeling of inner peace will be the result of permanent change.

- The other path is through rationalization, justifying the wrong. Rationalization is the result of low cognitive dissonance. The feeling of inner peace is only a temporary state; your reality will not have changed.

Chapter 4
The A-Gap Reality

∞

RREPS vs REPSS

A-Gap thinking is dominated by the preoccupation of struggle; that doing the right things are too difficult, too challenging, too painful, and too costly. Struggle scares the majority of people away from a challenge. An investment of time, energy, exertion, and money strikes fear into many hearts. The fear of struggle feeds the enemy of your state: excuses.

Chronic excuse-making is the product of *RREPS:*

- **R**epeated **R**ewarded **E**xcuses **P**roduce **S**oftness.

Excuses become hardwired when they are consistently rewarded and never challenged.

Excuse-making is caused by weakness and promotes more weakness. Excuses are the greatest limitation of potential and progress. Left unchecked, making up excuses and believing them becomes habitual until fiction obscures non-fiction, and reality can no longer be distinguished. Fear and reward are anabolic agents of excuses. As fear progresses, so do excuses. When excuses are rewarded, excuse-making turns into expertise. Fear and reward expand the scope and magnitude of excuses. Excuses are the only solution for those who are unwilling to try to solve a problem. Excuses are the quick fix. Excuses are cheap alternatives to working out problems. Excuses are not only attempts to deceive those around you, they are acts of self-deception. Self deception sabotages self.

Here's a test to help you establish the magnitude of your excuse-making: Record your dialogue for one hour, or one day, or one week. Listen to it and keep score. Identify the presence or absence of excuses when it's time to make a health-related decision about what to eat or when to exercise. Add them up and figure out if you are an excuse-making junkie or not.

It's impossible to get into top shape if you have an incredibly high tolerance for the pain of self-deception. The secret is to lower the pain threshold. It's worked for everyone I've coached who has put their mind to changing their lives. The moment they lowered their threshold for the *pain of being F'up*, they started losing fat. Mind fat first, followed by body fat.

Stop making excuses. Take ownership of the problem. Be honest.

Good news! There's a solution to habitual excuse-making.

The solution is *REPSS:*

- **R**ewarding **E**xtraordinary **P**erformance **S**trengthens & **S**ucceeds.

REPSS leads to *more* REPSS:

- **R**elieving **E**xtreme **P**ain **S**trengthens & **S**ucceeds

The difference between Strong Habits and Fat Habits is what gets rewarded. The reason why people fail to lose fat and quit trying is the failure to get rewarded for their accomplishments. There are two kinds of rewards: inner and outer, intrinsic and extrinsic. Inside rewards are the most powerful, hands down. There's no contest. Inside rewards are built to last, and they will make you built to last. The reasons are reliability and consistency. Inner rewards not only have the highest credibility, you can call them out anytime for as long as you want. Getting in shape is the intrinsic reward that leads to more REPSS (pain relief).

Conclusion: One *REP* leads to another *REP*:

- **R**ewarding **E**xtraordinary **P**erformance...
  Relieves **E**xtreme **P**ain

Mindset

Re-define "Extraordinary Performance"

We've been brainwashed to believe that there's a difference between ordinary and extraordinary performance. But, there isn't. There's no difference. That's why I remove the word "ordinary" from my coaching vocabulary. There is no such thing as ordinary. There is only extraordinary and mediocre, extraordinary and lazy, extraordinary and pitiful. But there's no "ordinary". Either you're trying your very best, or you're not. If you are trying you're very best, or *attempting to try your very best* by moving in that direction, your performance is extraordinary. If you're in the game and giving all you've got, your performance is extraordinary. But if you're dogging it, if you are not trying your very best, or even attempting to move in the direction of your very best, your performance is mediocre, or lazy, or pitiful. Not ordinary.

Every meaningful rep is an extraordinary accomplishment. A "meaningful rep" is defined as every single step you take toward getting in top shape. Every lift, every step of a run, every morsel of good food works toward top shape. All meaningful reps are extraordinary because *doing the right thing* is *always extraordinary.* The biggest mi take you can make in your fitness journey is to underestimate a meaningful rep. Never de-value even one step of your journey. Include "sticking-to-it" in your definition of "extraordinary performance." Grinding out every single rep, every step you take is epic. Nothing positive is ordinary. It's truly extraordinary to do the right things consistently because it is incredibly easy to do wrong. Each right step is a moral victory.

Re-define "Reward"

A big mistake in the fat-losing process is the expectation of immediate fat reward, that is, immediate gratification of achieving all fitness goals ASAP. Overnight. Breaking speed limits. That won't happen. Fat grows faster than it loses. If you are hooked on immediate gratification of the fattest reward possible, you will fail. Guaranteed.

Re-define "reward" to mean "the rush". The rush is the lifter's high; the "pump". The physical pump, intellectual pump, emotional pump, and spiritual pump of spilling your guts. The pump is an addictive feeling brought on by the adrenaline and mental rush of knowing you've just accomplished an extraordinary feat – beating the odds. The lifter's high is about reaching higher, and higher. You'll never get bored of the pump. The lifter's high is never monotonous.

The inner reward of the pump is incomparable. It's an escape from any hell. It fuels an inner fire, but only if you open your heart and mind to it. Otherwise, you'll miss it. Like all other sacred moments in life, if you're not paying attention, the sacred moment passes by unnoticed, because you're in a rush. Being in a rush misses the true rush. Nothing is more important to long-term fitness success than experiencing the reward of the lifter's high: winning the battle of the mind by eating right, exercising right, and doing both consistently. The lifter's high of not breaking down. The lifter's high of not giving up, and not giving in.

Define yourself as an "Athlete"
The athlete's mindset will prevent you from quitting. Anyone who competes in the daily grind against the strongest opponent, one's mind, is an "athlete". If you are in the game of fitness, you are an "athlete". Defining yourself as an athlete gives you higher purpose, and higher meaning. The athlete's mindset will stop you from quitting. The true athletic mindset never gives up, and never gives in. Never. Defining yourself as an athlete changes the focus of your fitness challenge by turning it into a *career*. Careers have staying power. A fitness career is one you'll never have to retire from. Fitness is for life. Defining yourself as an athlete is the turning point that leads to the turnaround and never turning back.

True athletes live for the intrinsic rewards. However, if you're an approval junkie, hooked on external rewards, your commitment to fitness and nutrition won't last, because external rewards are inconsistent and unreliable. They're fickle. You can't count on them. If you need to post pictures on Facebook and chronically check to see how many *likes* your picture received, you will be deceived. It won't work out. If you won't work out for yourself, it won't last.

Find a mentor

The mentor-protégé relationship is a powerful force of nature and nurture. A true mentor will not only appeal to your conscience, he/she will teach you how to do for yourself. A true mentor will make performance demands that guarantee success. It's impossible to fail in this type of relationship because it's based on the truth. If it *does* fail, if you *do not* achieve your goals, the relationship was not a true mentor-protégé one, it was only friendship.

The test of the mentor-protégé relationship is revealed in the interest-rate. Mentors have low self-interest but high interest in the protégé's development. They are obsessed with the development of the protégé; they see no goal except the development of the protégé. Mentors are not friends, not cheerleaders, and most importantly, not enablers. A true mentor has one mission: change your weakness into strength.

Make it your top priority to find a mentor. *A true mentor is the voice of your conscience.*

∞

Chapter 4 Summary

- A-gap thinking is excuse-making Excuses become chronic when they are consistently rewarded and never challenged.

- Change your mindset; redefine "extraordinary performance" and "reward."

- See yourself as an "athlete."

- Find a true mentor.